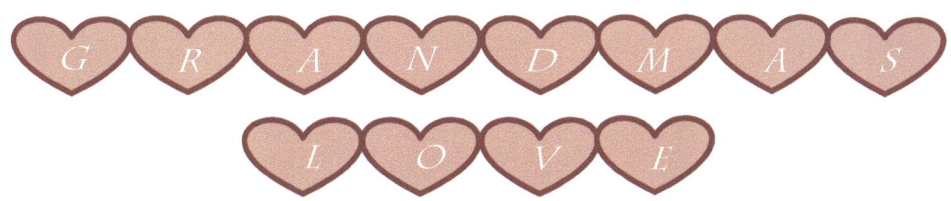

Grandmas are special.
They love forever.
No matter what.

You are always in their heart.
Even if they cannot remember your name,
They know you are theirs.
They still love you.
No matter what.

They held your hands when you were little.
Hold their hands when they grow old.
Keep them in your heart.
Never stop loving them.
Never forget them.
No matter what.

Clancy
Jasper

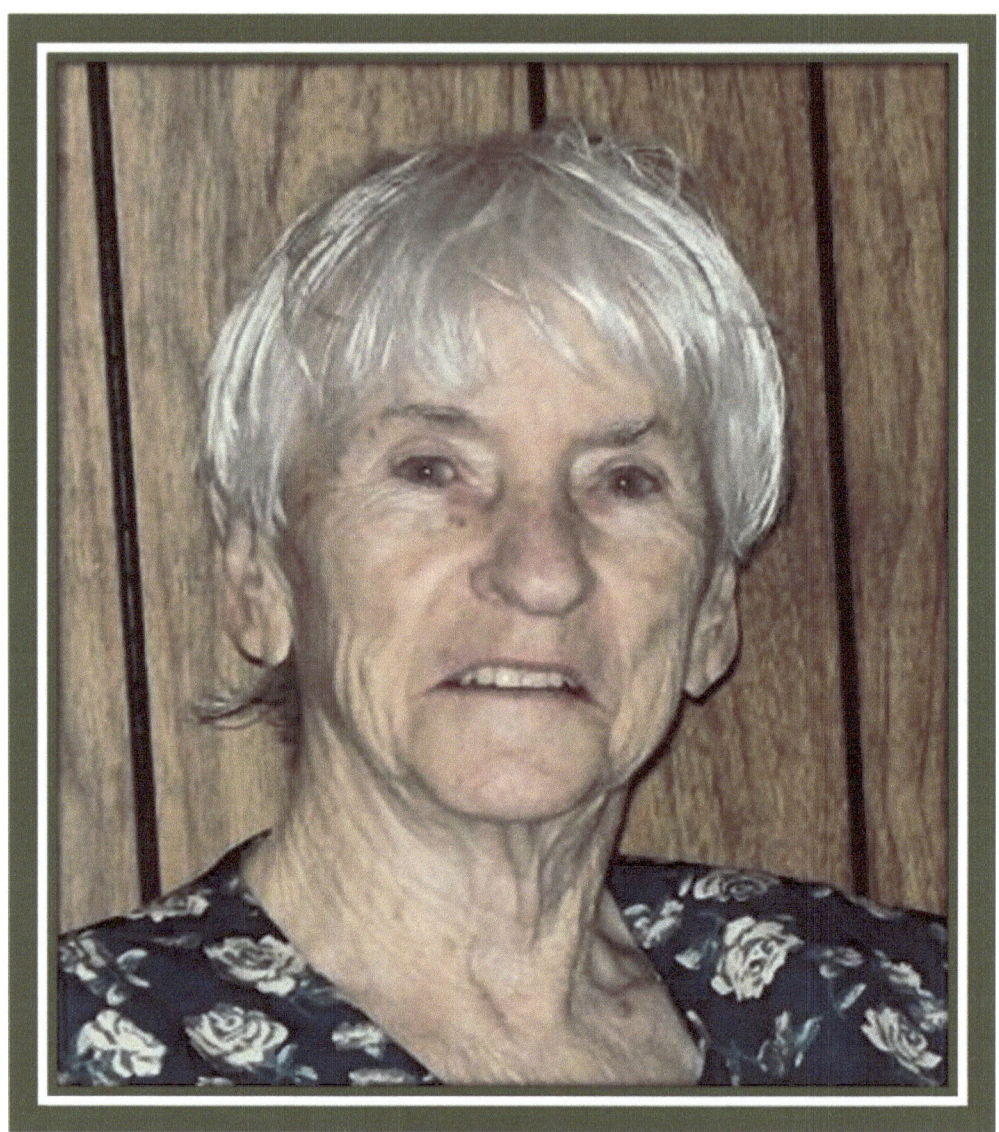

Claudia Jean Luttjohann
April 1, 1926 – November 29, 2012

Dear Grandma,
I hope you like my book.
I wrote it just for you.
I miss you.
Love,
Clancy Jasper

Did You Know My Grandma?

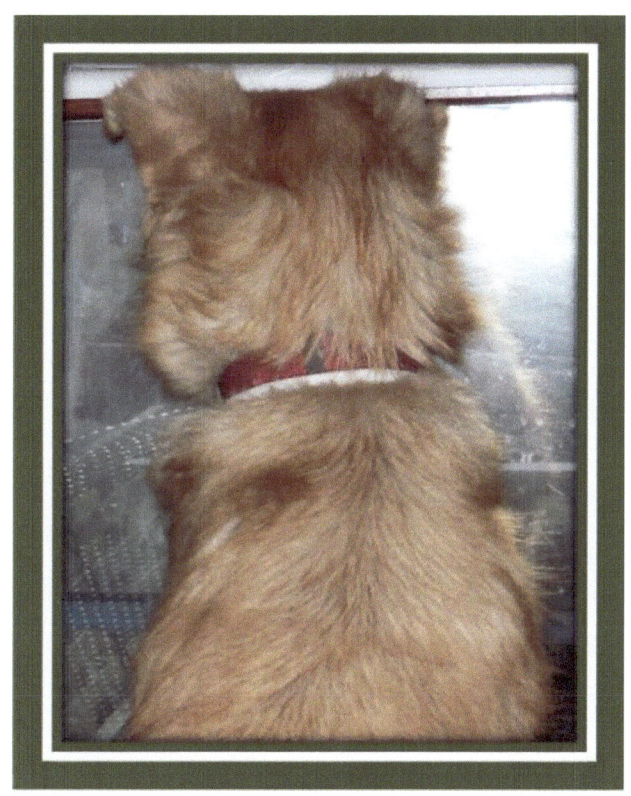

By
Clancy Jasper
and
Carol Luttjohann, MA, MSW

DEDICATION

For the best grandma ever,

MY GRANDMA,

Claudia Jean Luttjohann.

I love her and miss her.

--Clancy Jasper—

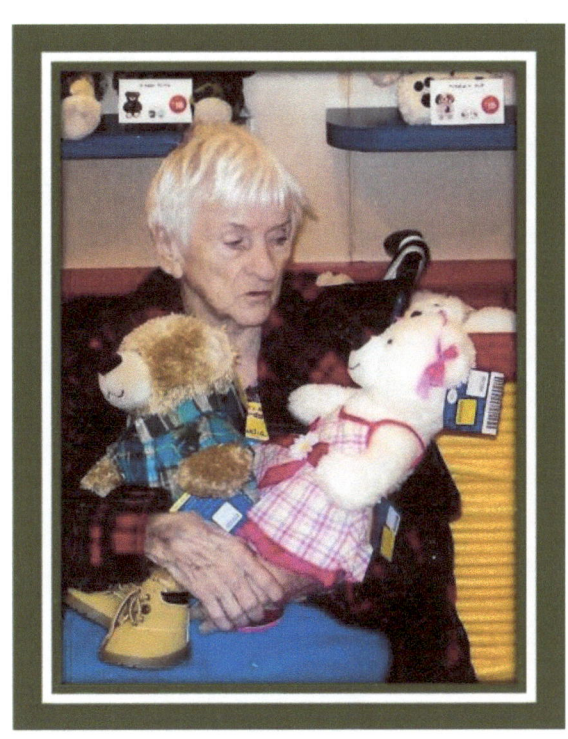

ACKNOWLEDGEMENTS

Thanks to my mom, Carol Luttjohann, I wrote this book. She helped a lot. My paws are too big for the keyboard. I told her what to write, and she wrote the words. She also had to check my spelling so if you find any mistakes, tell Mom.

And thanks to Aunt Deanna Miles and Aunt Chris Harvey for reading it and telling me how good it is. They are my aunts. They have to say it's good.

All of them love Grandma, too.

ABOUT GRANDMA CLAUDIA

Claudia Luttjohann was fortunate to be able to remain in her own house at the end of her life. Her daughter, Carol, and their pets, Clancy Jasper, a Border Collie mix, and Delilah Lucille, a calico cat, cared for Claudia.

This book is about Clancy's interactions with his grandma Claudia. There are pictures of Claudia throughout the time Clancy and Carol cared for her – from the early days through her final days. Not all of the pictures go with the stories, but they are pictures that show Clancy's special relationship with his Grandma.

Clancy was very protective of Claudia. They bonded the moment they met. He definitely feels the loss of his grandma. He also is a wonderful companion and comfort for Carol.

It is the hope that these stories and poems will provide some laughter and comfort to others who have lost their very special grandma.

The First Time I Saw Grandma

Mom said she saw an ad in a newspaper for free puppies. The ad said the puppies were half Border Collie. Mom knows Border Collies are smart, and one would be a good dog to help her take care of her mom – my grandma.

Mom and Grandma had to go on a pretty long drive to see me. But they did. When they came into the house, Mom came over and picked me up.

She was nice, but I kept looking at Grandma. I knew she was special. And I knew Mom needed help with Grandma, and I was just the dog for the job.

Then Mom put me on the floor so she could look at my brothers. They all ran the other way. Our dog-mom came into the room, and they wanted to nurse. I was hungry, but I wanted to stay with Mom and Grandma.

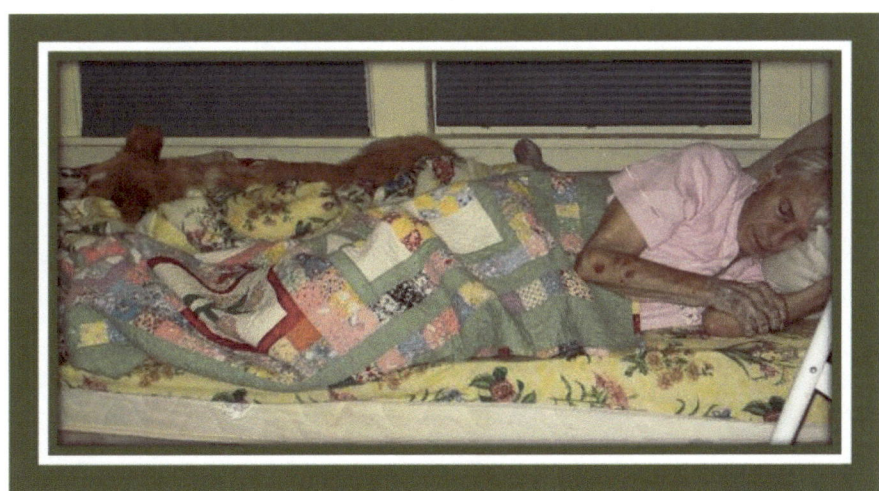

Mom decided to take me home. When the three of us got in the truck, she gave me to Grandma to hold.

I snuggled up to her, and she sang songs to me. She sang something about rocking a baby and something about shoes. I was not sure about rocks and babies, but I was kind of interested in the shoes. I thought they might be good to chew. But instead I fell asleep.

I loved to snuggle with my grandma. She loved me to snuggle with her. I would lick her face sometimes. She liked that. I liked the taste of ice cream on her face.

Silly Grandma Kisses Are Good

Grandma was sitting in her chair.
I decided to give her some kisses.
She got tired of kisses and covered her head.
I said, "Oh, good!
Now we are playing hide and seek.
Where's Grandma?"
Mom laughed.

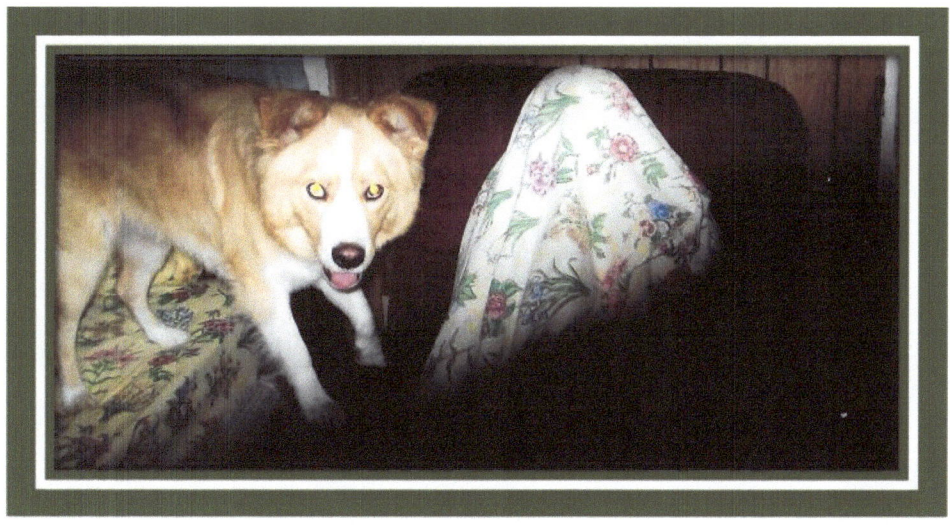

Grandma Said, "Apologize To My Dog!"

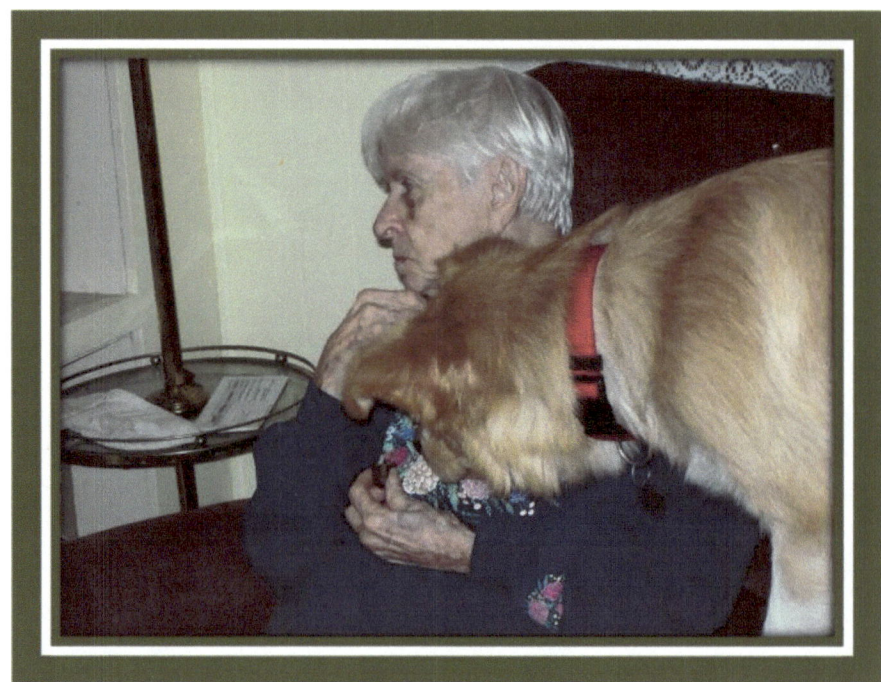

Mom was sitting in the pink chair eating. I wanted something to eat, too, so I jumped on the bed beside her and watched her very carefully. I leaned over to get a closer look.

Mom put her arm in front of me so I wouldn't eat her supper.

Grandma thought Mom hit me. She said, "Apologize to my dog!"

I laughed.

Another day I jumped on Mom's foot. She said, "Ow! That hurt! Dang dog!"

Grandma said, "Don't talk to my dog like that. Apologize to my dog."

Grandma and I were special buddies.

We took care of each other.

Mom loves Grandma, and Grandma loves Mom, too. I love both of them!

I miss Grandma saying, "Apologize to my dog!"

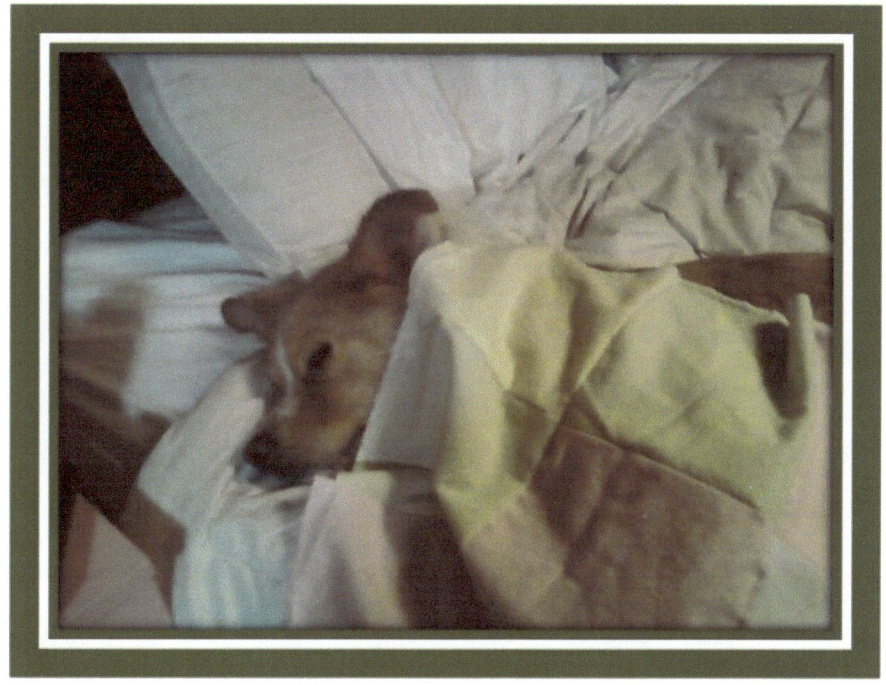

Mom's Favorite Video

One day Grandma was eating mashed potatoes, spinach, baked beans, and lentils. She told Mom she would not eat until I got a plate, too. So Mom gave me a plate of mashed potatoes, spinach, and lentils. She would not give me any baked beans.

Grandma let me clean off her plate She sat and watched me eat. She let me eat baked beans. She pushed the food around on the plate to make it easier for me to reach.

I jumped down out of my chair and went over by Grandma. She said, "You are such a good dog." Then she started to sing to me.

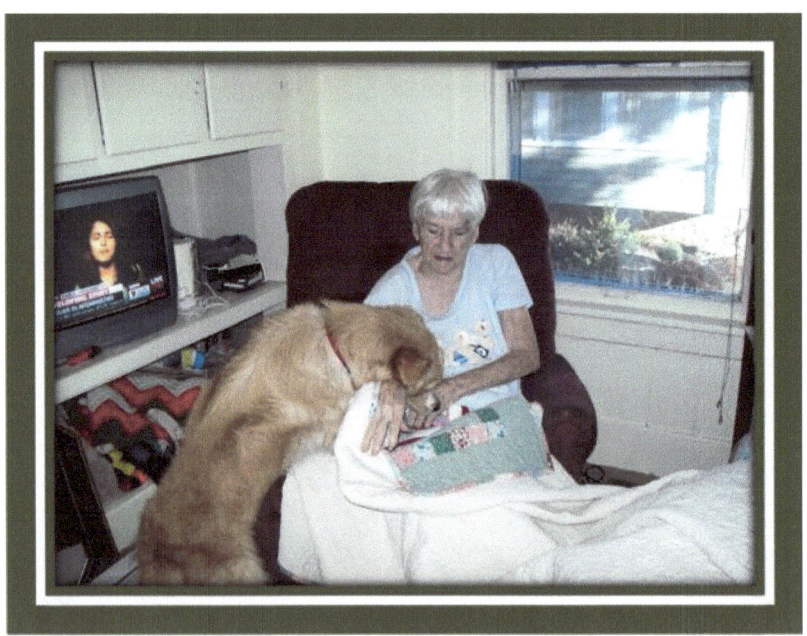

She fed me with her spoon. Then she decided to eat some more. She picked up her plate and started eating. So I jumped on the bed beside her, and we shared her food.

She used a spoon, and I helped myself. She patted my head and told me I was a good dog.

Grandmas are so special. And I had the best.

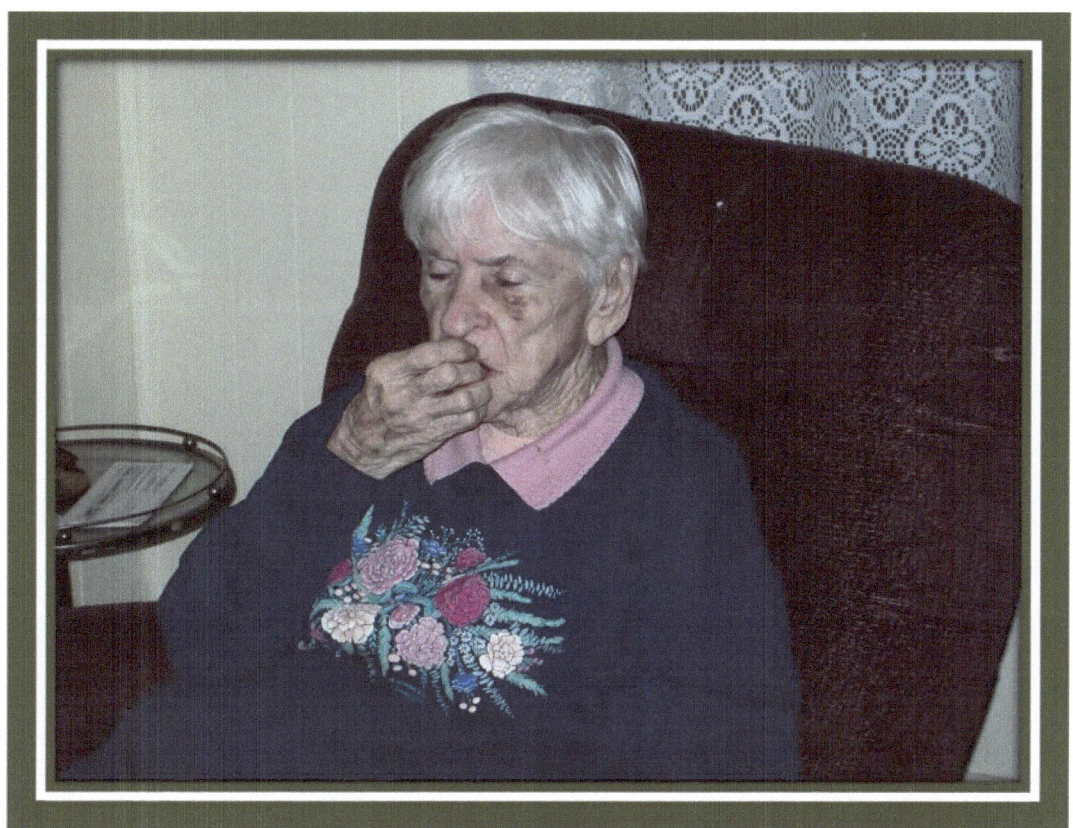

Do you see Grandma's eye? One day I got really excited and jumped on the bed and bumped her. That is how she got the black eye. Grandma said, "That's okay, Honey. You didn't mean to do that." That's what Grandmas do. They say everything is okay.

My Favorite Tree

There is a big tree in my backyard. I love that tree. Mom and Grandma would do silly things. I would laugh. Sometimes I would laugh and would almost not make it to my favorite tree..

Once Mom made some shelves for the back porch. Grandma and I were inside, but the cat, Delilah, was on the porch.

Mom bumped the shelves on the fan. They started to fall. Delilah was bouncing around. She looked like a furry ping pong ball. I ran to my tree.

Mom was looking for her cell phone. She looked under the bed. She looked under Grandma's bed. She took things out of drawers. She moved stuff.

Finally she found it in her pocket.

Another trip to the tree for me.

Catching Flies

"There are lot of flies in here, and they are bothering Grandma," Mom said. She was swatting flies, but it scared Grandma. So she stopped.

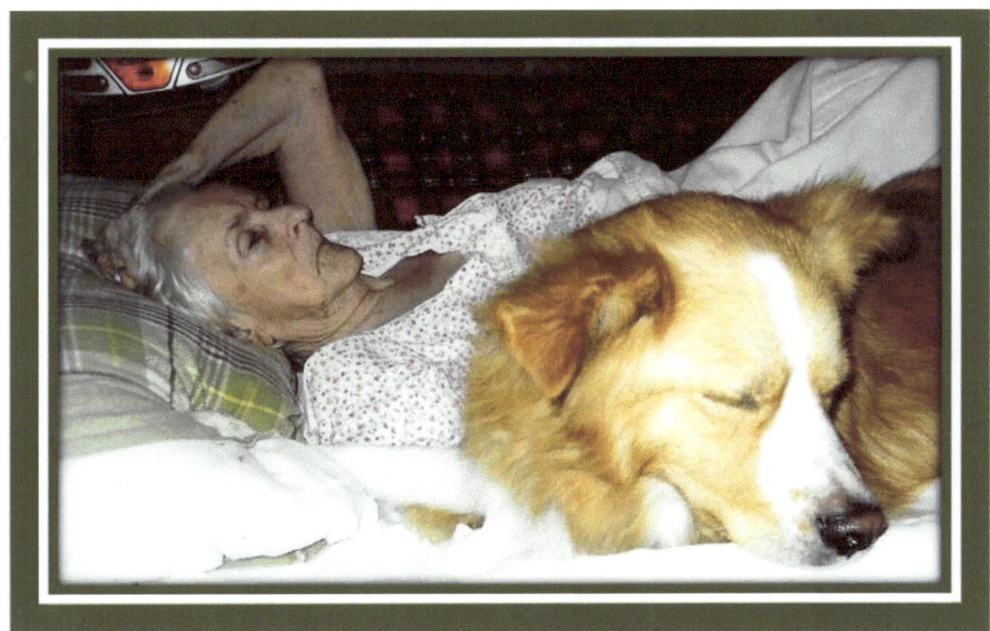

But the flies did not stop. I had to do something. So I jumped on Grandma's bed and laid down at the very top of it above her head. I snapped at flies that came by her. I caught a lot. It took me a while, but I got them all.

Then Grandma and I took a nap on her bed.

Toes

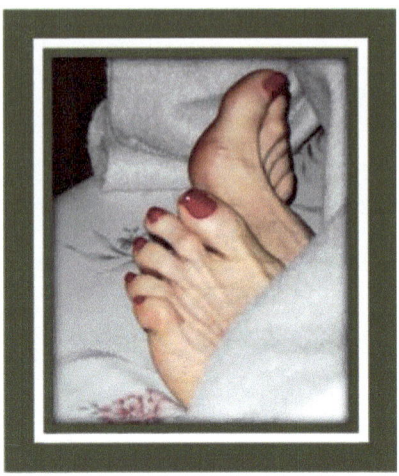

One day, Sara, one of Grandma's aides, said she was going to paint Grandma's nails. First, I had to figure out nails.

Mom used nails to build things. I was wondering, "Did Mom build Grandma with nails?" It was very confusing.

Then I learned people have things on their fingers and toes they call nails. I have no idea why, but that is what they call them.

Anyway, Sara, was painting them. That means she had a tiny bottle with some paint in it and used a really, really small brush and put the colored stuff on Grandma's nails – the ones on her fingers and toes.

Sara told Grandma, "You are going to look so pretty."

Grandma said, "I am pretty."

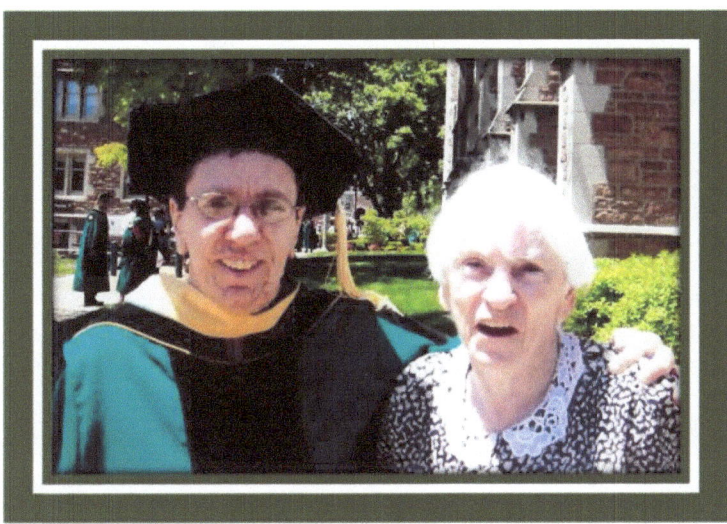

This is Mom and Grandma at Mom's graduation from Washington University in St Louis. Mom drove to Topeka and took Grandma back to watch. Grandma loved being there to see her daughter graduate.

Grandma was beautiful – not just her nails and hair and stuff like that. Grandma was a beautiful person in ways it really counts.

She was funny and nice and loved people and took care of her friends and family and loved being alive.

Did You Know My Grandma?

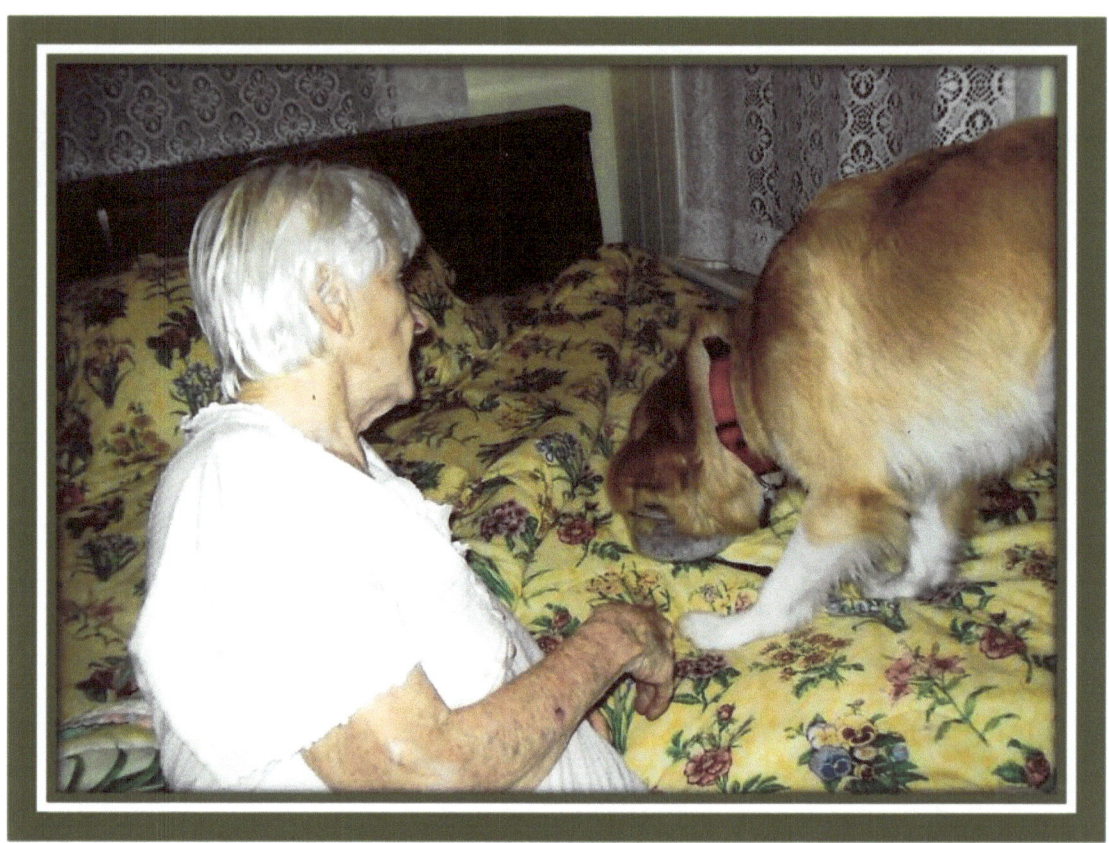

My grandma shared ice cream with me.

My Grandma let me eat off of her plate.

Most of the time.

Did you know my grandma?

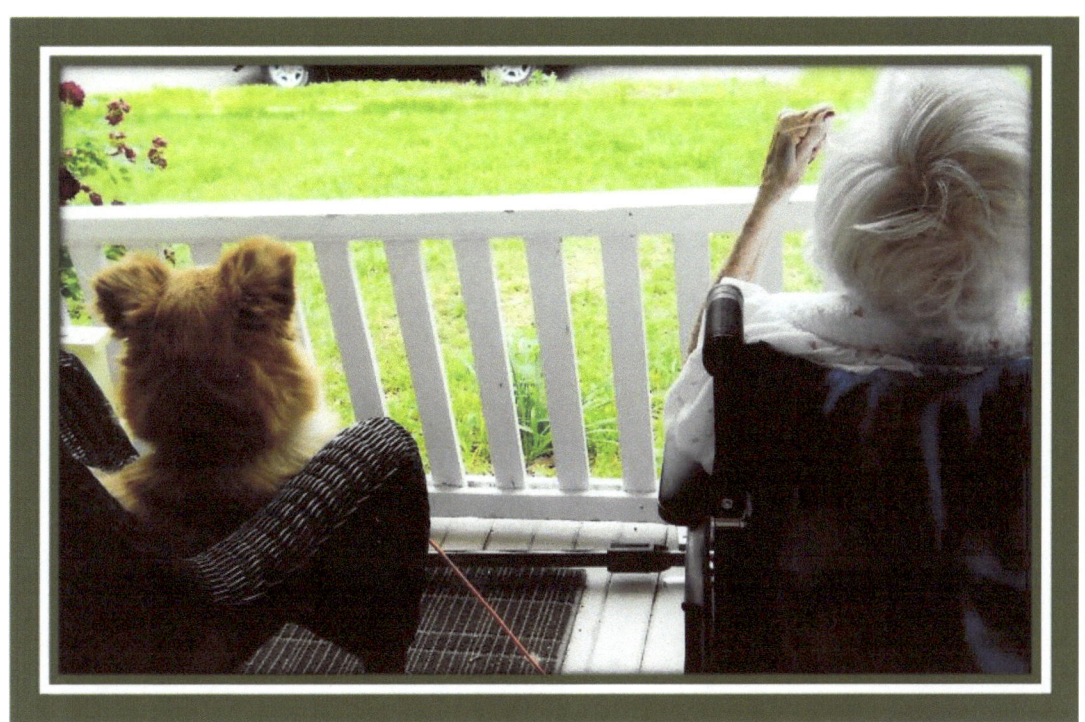

My grandma liked to go for walks with me and Mom.

My grandma and I liked to sit on the porch.

We each had our own chair.

Did you know my grandma?

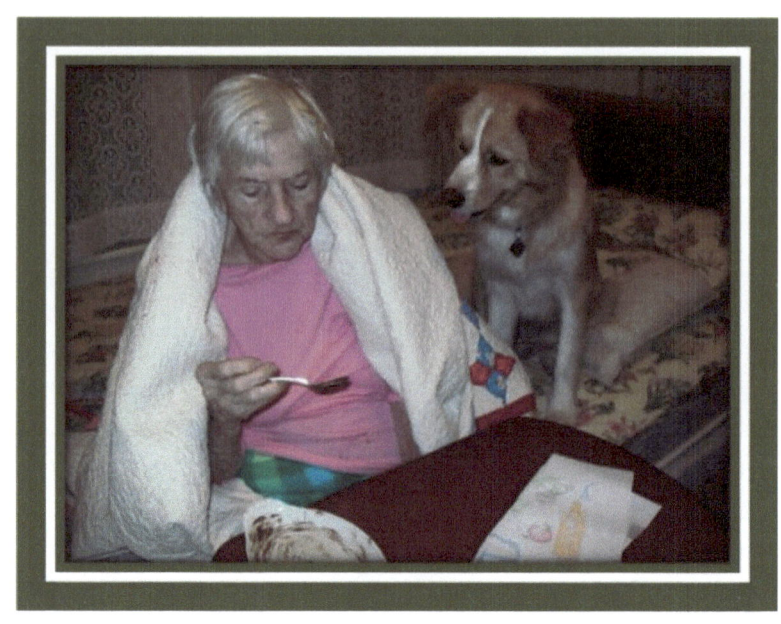

My grandma made Mom apologize to me a lot.

Did you know my grandma?

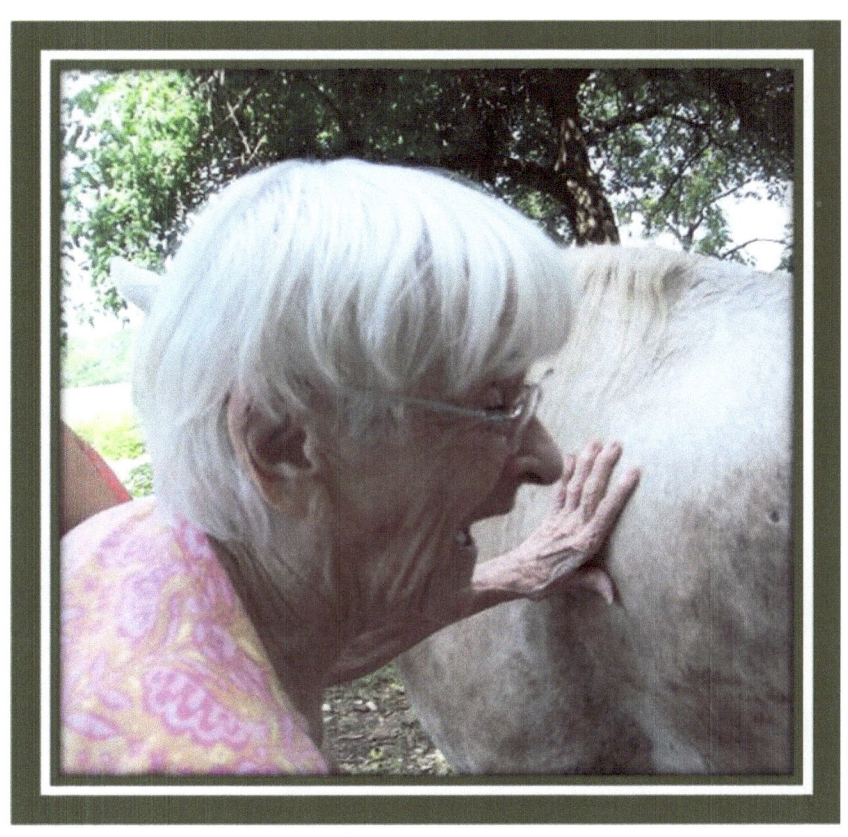

My grandma loved all kinds of animals

She told me to be especially nice to rabbits.

Rabbits are dogs, too.

Did you know my grandma?

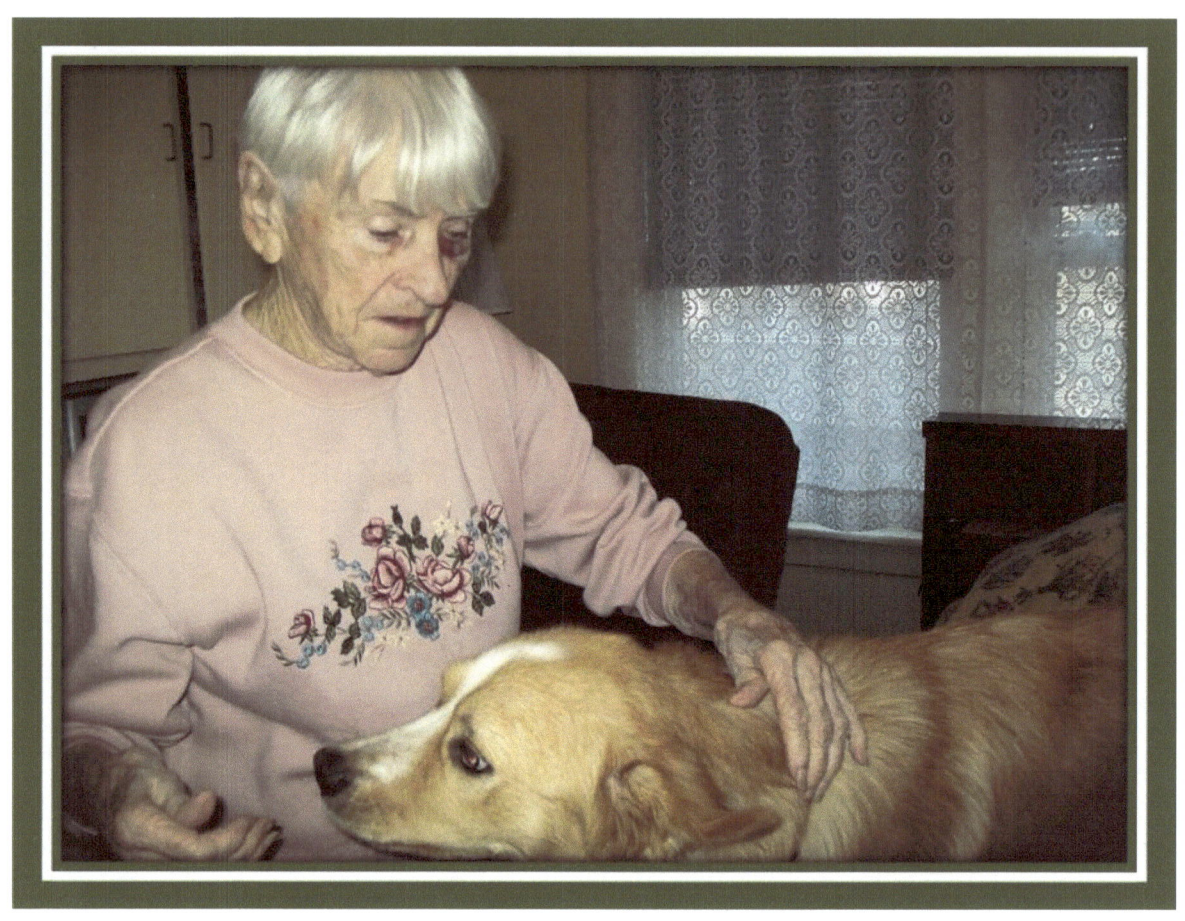

My grandma would get upset when I barked a lot.

Sometimes.

Did you know my grandma?

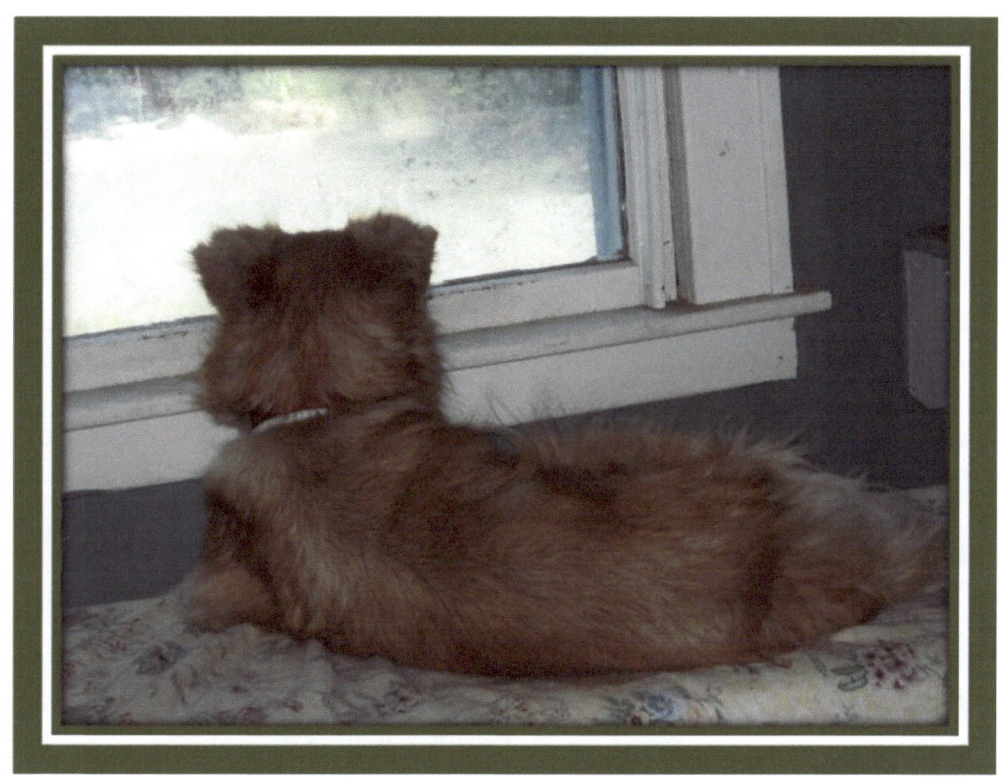

My grandma loves me.

I love Grandma.

Did you know my grandma?

Eating Ice Cream With Grandma
In Ten Easy Steps

1.

Get a pretty big bowl out of the cabinet. It has to hold ice cream for three. Grandma eats enough for two. Maybe it should be enough to hold ice cream for four so we can each eat half.

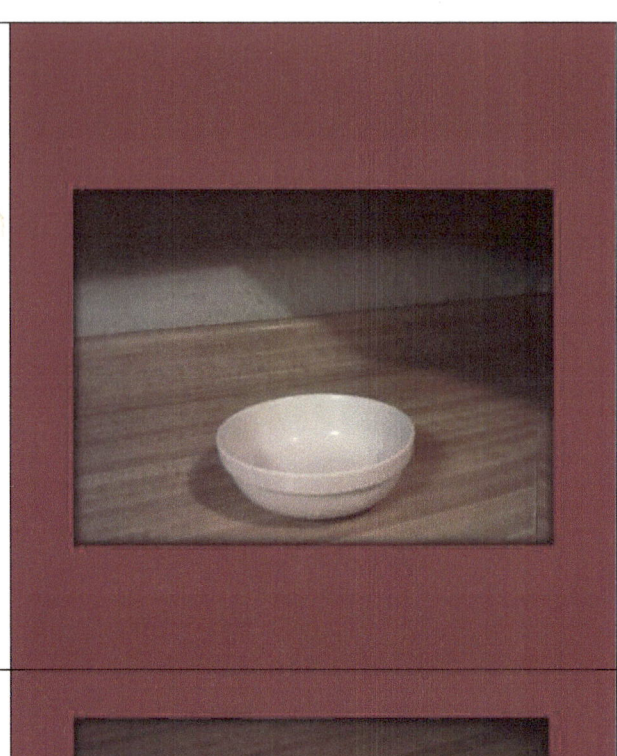

2.

Get the ice cream scoop and two spoons out of the drawer.

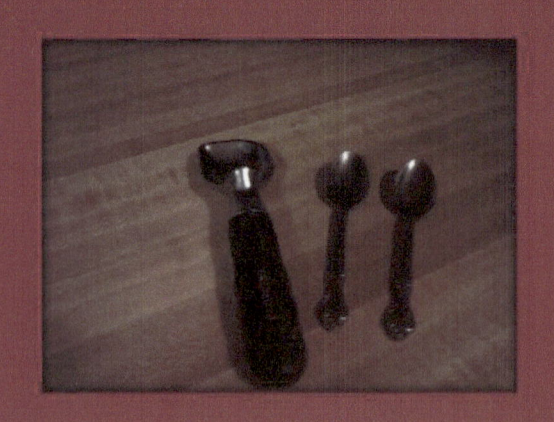

3.

Get the ice cream out of the freezer. It doesn't matter what kind. Grandma eats all kinds.

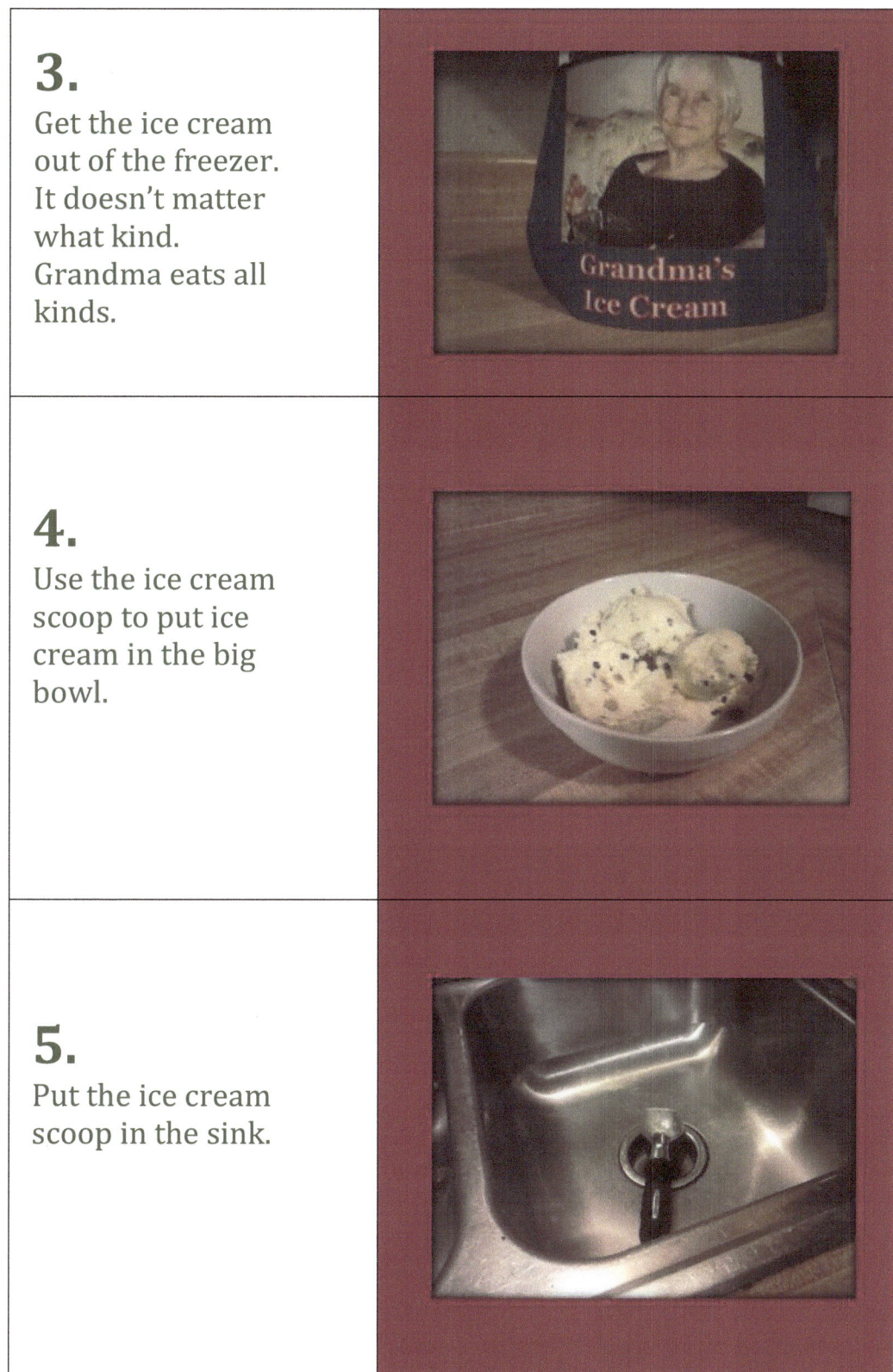

4.

Use the ice cream scoop to put ice cream in the big bowl.

5.

Put the ice cream scoop in the sink.

6.

Put the ice cream back in the freezer.

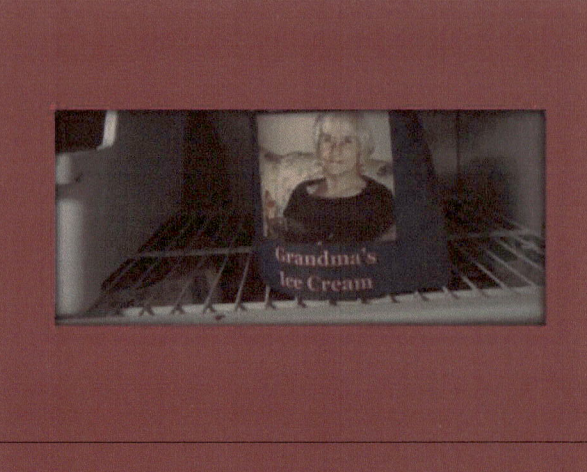

7.

Give Grandma her ice cream and two spoons. She is supposed to use one to eat with and one to feed me.

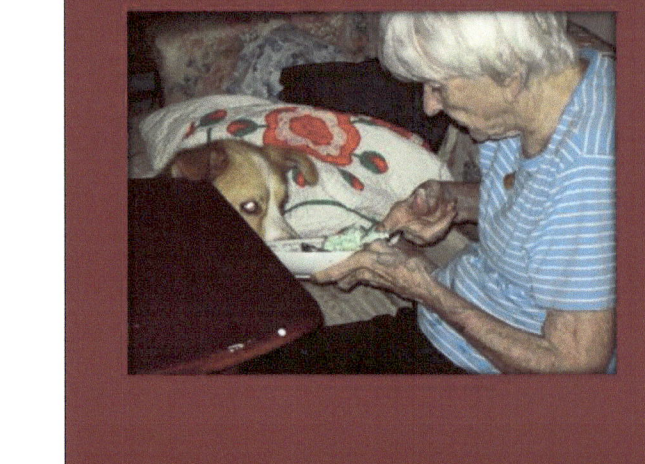

8.

Watch Grandma eat ice cream. Wiggle tail and whimper so she knows I am waiting for some. Staring at food will get sympathy.

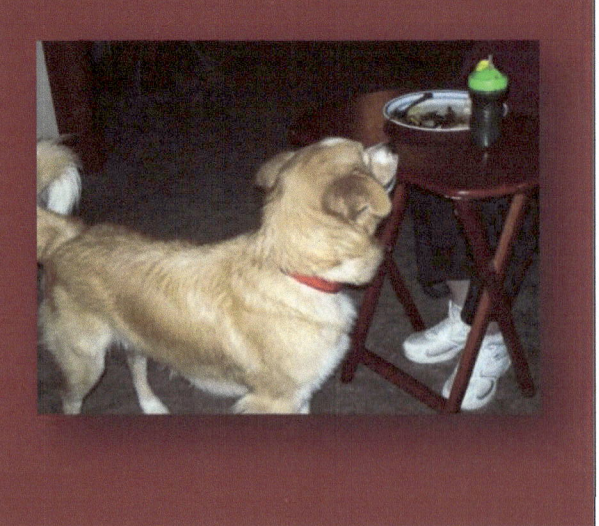

9.

Put paws on Grandma's lap and eat ice cream from bowl. She will use her spoon. She obviously forgot to share.

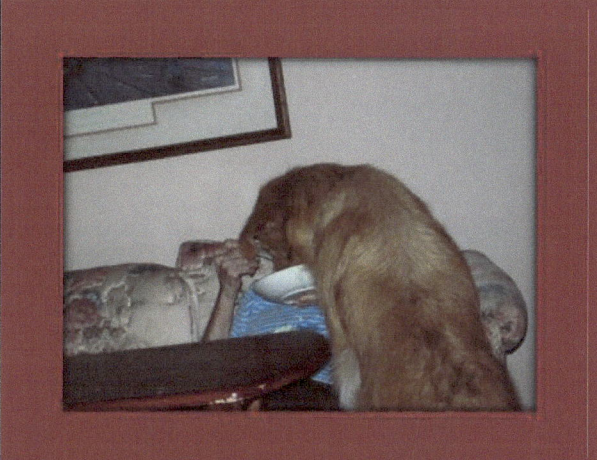

10.

Clean all the leftover ice cream off of Grandma. Shoes are a good place to check.

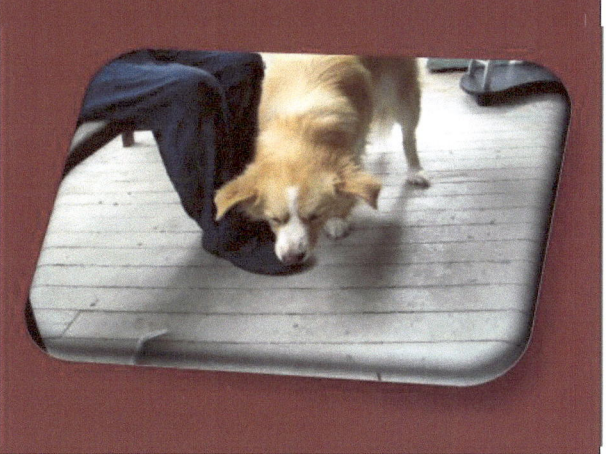

So Special

When I was a baby, my grandma held me. She sang songs, and she rocked me. She took good care of me.

Then when she had trouble doing things she used to do, it was my job to help her.

Mom fed Grandma and helped keep her clean. She cooked for Grandma. And I got to eat everything, too. That was Grandma's rule.

Sometimes things were really hard for Mom.

Then I had both of them to take care of. That was okay.

I love Mom and Grandma.

I knew the very first time I saw Grandma she was special.

And I was right.

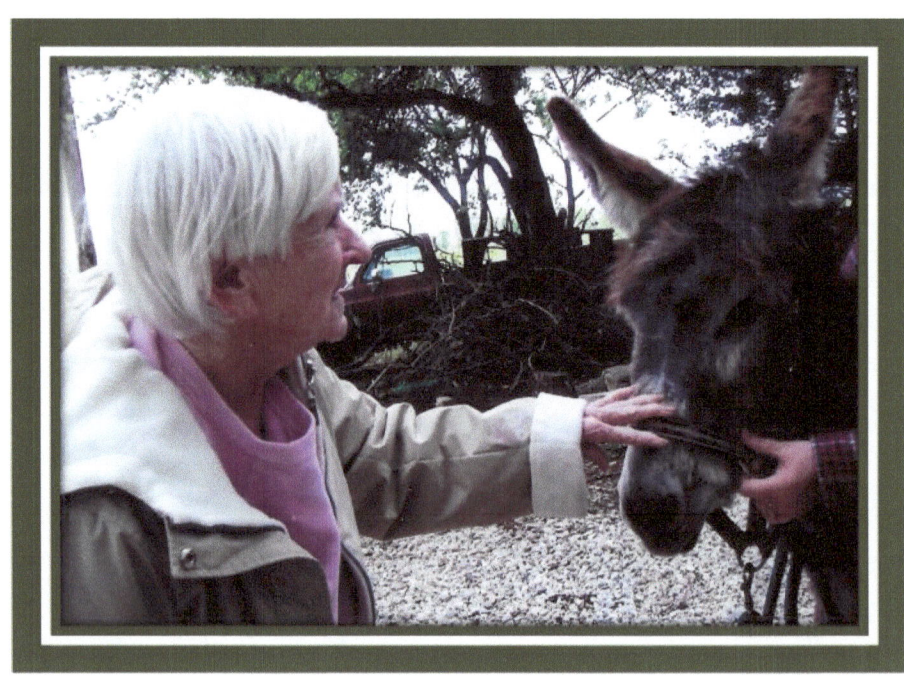

Grandma Claudia Is Mine

Grandmas are special people.
They love grandkids and grand-dogs and even grand-cats.

Grandma Claudia could look at my mouth and
know what I was hungry for.
Usually ice cream.

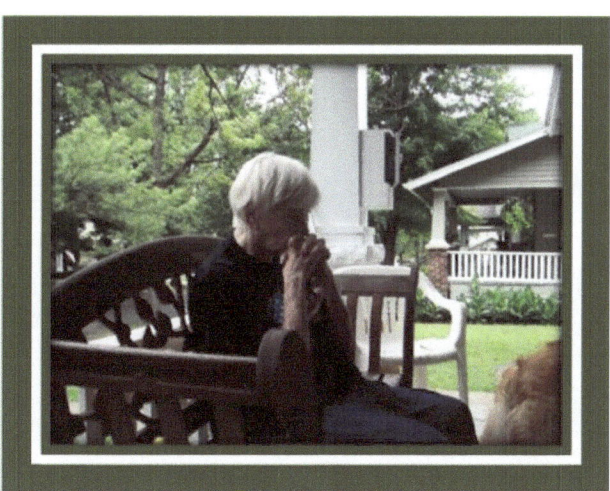

Grandma Claudia gave the best hugs.
She even hugged my sister, Delilah, the cat.
Grandma Claudia prayed for my mom and me.

Grandma Claudia told me I was special
Lots of grandmas do that stuff
But Grandma Claudia is mine.

I Can't Find Grandma

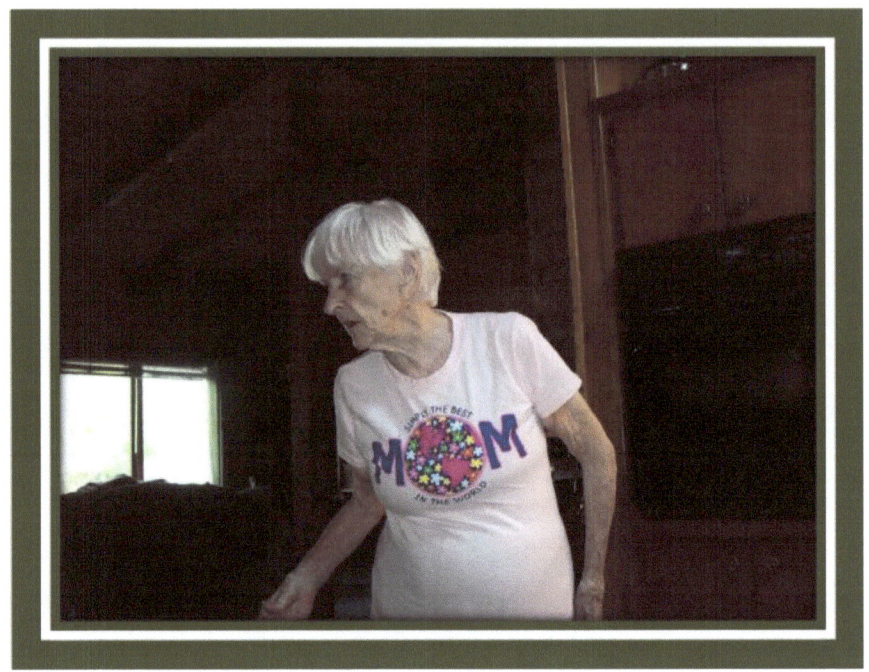

I can smell her

I know she has been here

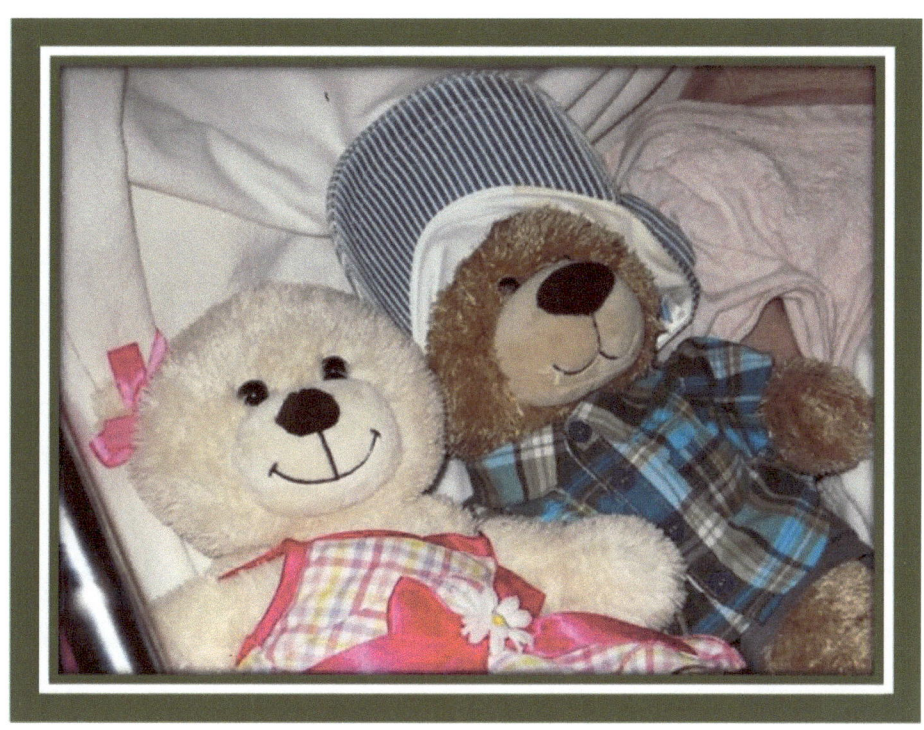

Her teddy bears are here
She loved her bears
She left them here with me and Mom

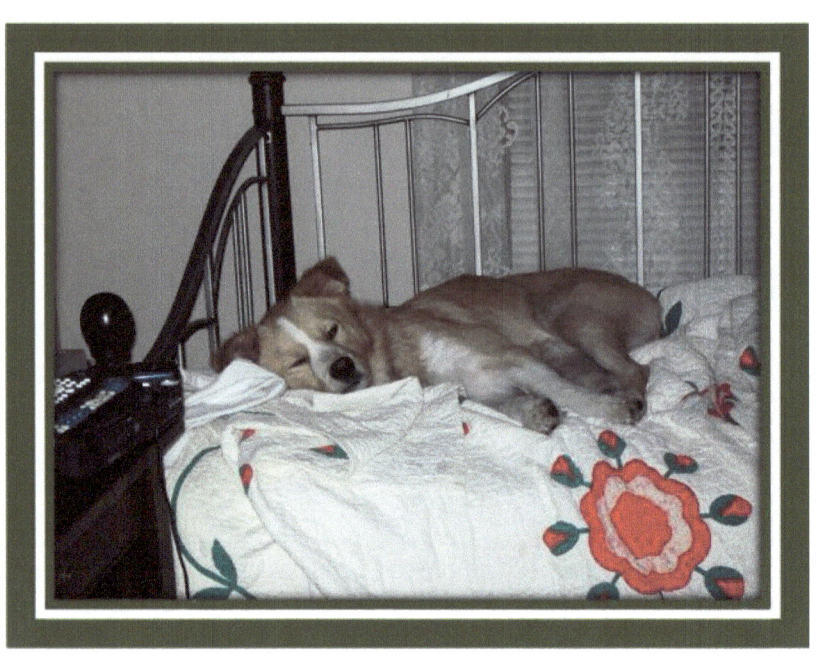

She used to sleep on her bed in the living room
Mom and I slept on Mom's bed
Sometimes I slept with Grandma

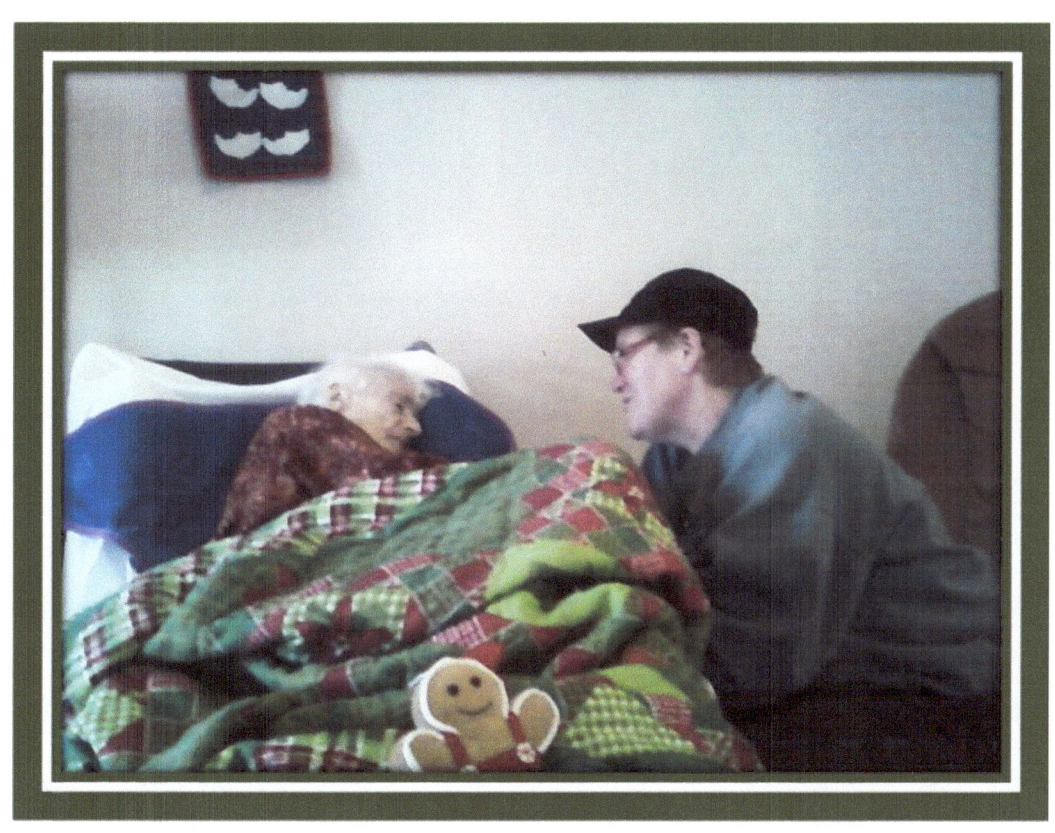

Grandma loved to sing.
Mom played lots of music for her.
Grandma liked Bing Crosby and Statler Brothers.
She liked John Denver, too.
She used to like Peter, Paul, and Mary.
Then one day she told Aunt Deanna,
"I've had enough of Peter, Paul, and what's her name?"

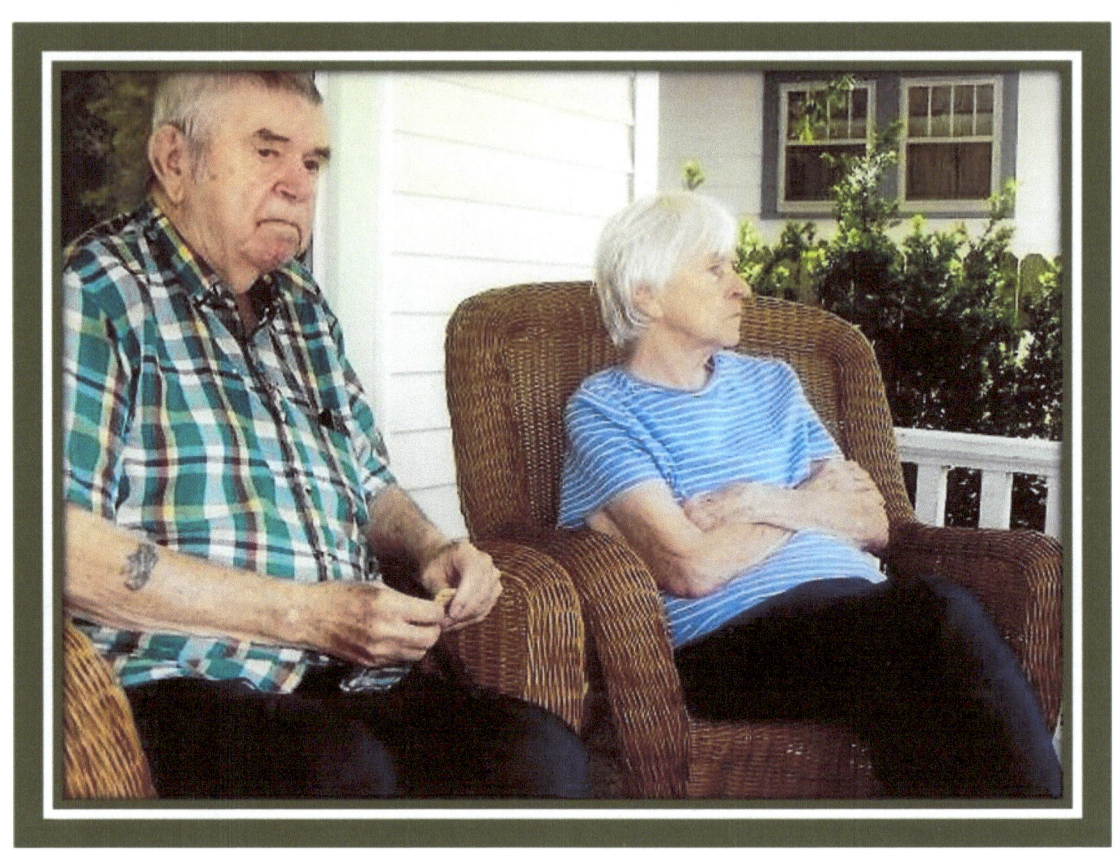

Mom said Grandma and Grandpa are together in heaven.
I guess that is okay.
Grandma and Grandpa love each other a lot
They were married almost 66 years
That's even more than I am in dog's years

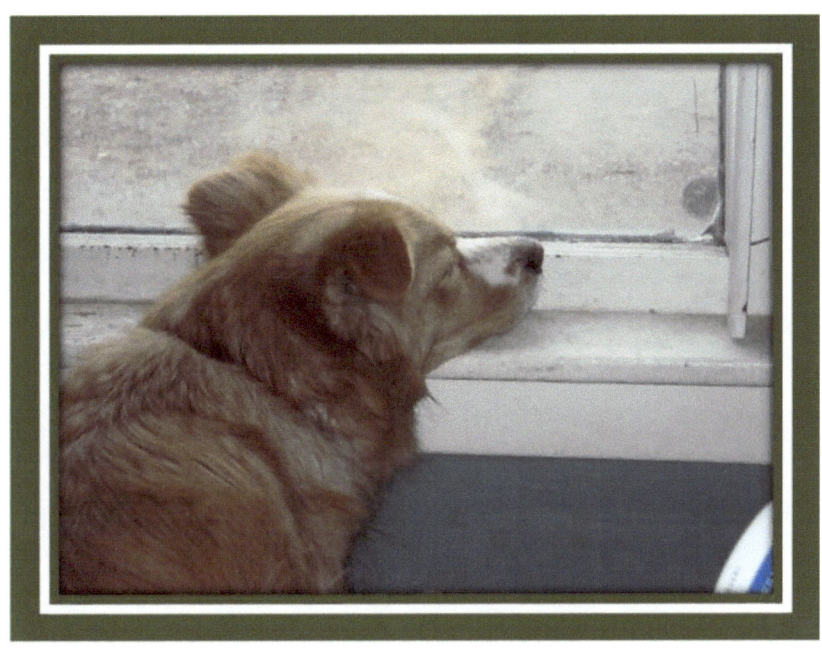

Grandma liked me to give her kisses good night
I liked giving her kisses
I miss Grandma

ABOUT THE AUTHOR

Carol Luttjohann earned her Bachelor of Arts at Ottawa University in Ottawa, Kansas, her Master of Arts in Religious Education at Southwestern Baptist Theological Seminary, and her Master of Social Work at Washington University in St. Louis.

After graduating from Washington University, she returned to Topeka to care for her parents. Carol lives in Topeka, Kansas with her dog, Clancy Jasper, and cat, Delilah Lucille.

She is active in advocating for and educating about people with dementia and for services for elderly to remain in their own homes. She is in the process of a startup non-profit, My Mother's Daughter, which will focus on services to elderly and caregivers to keep people in their own homes.

She can be reached by email at ClaudiasPlace@gmx.com or on her blog at http://carolluttjohann.wordpress.com

OTHER BOOKS BY CAROL LUTTJOHANN

She's Not An Old Lady With Dementia She's My Mother

One Day At A Time For Caregivers (March 2014)

Discovering Pineapple (2014)

Carol's books are (will be) available on Amazon.com